Homemade Lotions and Body Butter

15 DIY Recipes for Organic Skin Care

Table of Contents

Introduction

The skin is the largest organ and it requires a lot of attention in order to stay healthy. One of the biggest threats is represented by dehydration, which becomes an even bigger issue to consider during the cold winter season. When the skin suffers from dehydration, it becomes dry and has an aged-aspect.

Store-bought products can be used to hydrate the skin but they do not even begin to compare to homemade lotions and body butters. These contain only natural, organic ingredients and they deliver a feeling of safety, as you will know exactly the product you are applying at the level of the skin.

Preparing homemade lotions and body butters is not as complicated as you might expect, especially if you will follow the recipes that have been included in this book. As you will have the opportunity to see for yourself, these recipes have a number of ingredients that you will have to gather, such as the nourishing oils, emulsifiers and essential oils (fragrances).

These recipes follow a basic pattern, in which you are first required to melt the nourishing oils & emulsifiers, adding the essential oils and other ingredients after the mixture has cooled down.

Before you move on to the first chapter and dive into the world of homemade skin care products, it is important to understand the difference between lotions and body butters. The first contain less nourishing butters, being made with water.

As for the body butters, these are made exclusively from butters, having a thicker consistency. When you are interested in a product that will hydrate your skin, without being too heavy or greasy, you will go with a lotion. On the other hand, during the winter, a body butter might be more suitable, as it will hydrate and nourish the skin at the same time.

You can also prepare lotion/butter bars, using muffin tins or silicone molds for such purposes. These have the advantage of being rubbed directly on the skin, offering an intensely hydrating effect.

As you will have the chance to see below, these are prepared exactly as regular lotions or body butters, with the exception of the final step, when they are poured into a silicone mold and placed in the fridge in order to harden.

No matter if you decide to prepare regular lotions/body butters or go with the bar version, it is guaranteed that you will have lots of fun. You will unleash your inner creativity and, as you will gain experience, you will diversity and customize the recipes included in this book.

Chapter 1 – Homemade lotions basics

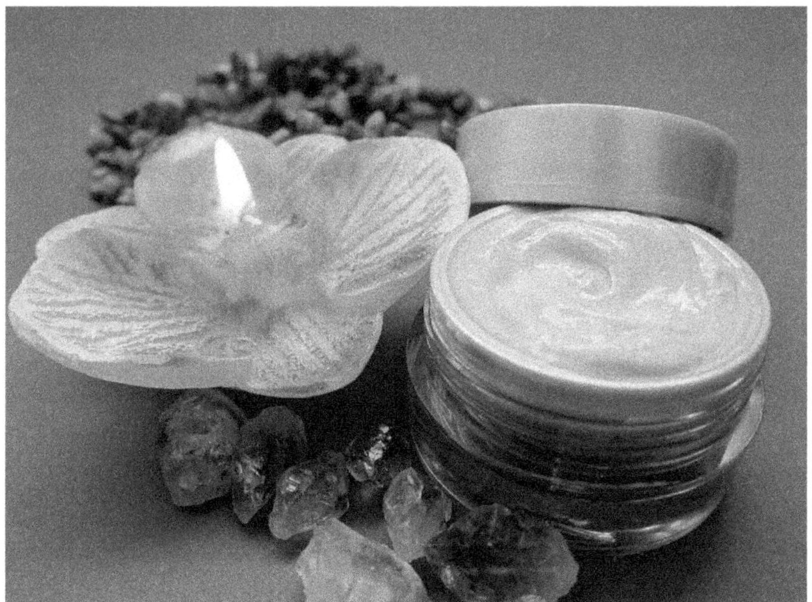

If you were to read the label of a store-bought lotion, you would see that it contains many chemicals and other potentially-harmful substances. In such situations, it is only normal that you are interested in creating your own lotion or body butter.

Like many other experiences in life, once you manage to make your first lotion, you won't have anything else to fear. In this chapter, we will introduce you into the wonderful world of homemade lotions and body butters. Find out everything you need to know before moving on to the actual recipes.

All homemade lotions & body butters recipes have a basic pattern and, once you grasp that, you can customize your recipes as you desire. First and foremost, it is highly important that you use the correct quantities, as this will ensure a stable product.

The texture of the lotion/body butter depends on the quantity you have used for each of the chosen ingredients; it is also influenced by the chosen emulsifier, co-emulsifier and essential oils. In some recipes, it is possible to use a number of additional ingredients, such as glycerin or fragrances.

As you will have the opportunity to see for yourself, there are certain ingredients that are found in all of the recipes. Among the most common ingredients, there are: coconut oil, shea butter, sweet almond oil, avocado oil and beeswax. Sweet almond oil can also be used for lightweight recipes, as it hydrates the skin, without leaving it greasy.

Avocado oil, on the other hand, is considered a medium-weight oil, which means that it will hydrate the skin more intensively (however, it is just as easily absorbed into the skin).

Shea butter is well known for its softness and also for its moisturizing properties. If added to a lotion or a body butter, it will guarantee a thicker consistency for the respective product. It also worth mentioning that it is a heavy-weight product, which means that it will leave the skin feeling a little bit greasy.

Nevertheless, it is absorbed into the skin and it does wonders when it comes to hydrating the skin. Coconut oil has similar properties, hydrating the skin and preventing the water loss at the level of the dry skin. Often used as an ingredient of homemade lotions and body butters, coconut oil is appreciated not only because of its moisturizing properties but also because of its delicious smell.

Emulsifiers are used in homemade lotions and body butters, in order to ensure the success of a product. They are the ones that allow for the ingredients to bind, contributing to the stability of the respective lotion.

Sometimes, co-emulsifiers are added to the same recipe, so as to guarantee a thicker, cream-like consistency of the product. One of the most common used emulsifiers in homemade lotions and body butters is beeswax; this can be purchased in a larger piece and then grated or directly available as pellets.

A homemade lotion or body butter would not be anything without the usage of essential oils. These are the ones that give out the scent of the product in question and the good news is that you can combine different fragrances for the same lotion or body butter.

Among the most commonly used essential oils, you will find the following: peppermint, lavender, lemon, orange, cinnamon, rosemary, carrot seed, chamomile, cranberry seed, Frankincense, myrrh, grapefruit, jasmine, lemongrass, rose, rosehip, sage, sandalwood, tea tree, valerian and ylang-ylang.

When you make a homemade lotion/body butter, as you gain experience, you have the opportunity to play with different recipes and add new ingredients. For example, you can create a chocolate body butter by adding cocoa butter into the mix. Or, if you are interested in a lotion with detoxifying properties, you can use matcha (green tea) powder.

Many more other ingredients can be added for color and texture, with fruits standing at the top of the list. Cranberries, grapes, peaches, grapefruits and lemons can be added to homemade lotions. You can also use fresh fruit juice, herbs and even apple cider vinegar. The choice is yours!

If you are looking for a unique alternative to lotions and body butters, you could always try preparing lotion/butter bars. These are prepared in a similar manner and using the same ingredients as regular lotions/body butters, with the difference being in being poured into silicone molds.

So, instead of pouring the mixture into a glass jar, you use silicone molds and place them in the fridge to harden. Lotion/butter bars can be rubbed directly on the skin, having equal moisturizing properties. Plus, they make quite nice gifts to offer to your someone special.

In case you are still wondering why should you be interested in preparing such body lotions/butters, keep in mind that such a product can nourish your skin and provide it with everything required. The ingredients chosen for these recipes are 100% natural, hydrating and rejuvenating the skin.

Depending on the chosen ingredients, you can even repair the damaged skin, by using a homemade lotion or body butter. Plus, you cannot deny the comfort you will obtain, knowing exactly the ingredients of such a product (you cannot say the same thing about a store-bought product).

In regard to the equipment, do not be too stressed, as you will not require as many items as you probably expect.

The list of recommended equipment includes the following: ceramic bowls, saucepan, glass jar(s), spatula, mixer (stand/hand), food processor/blender, silicone molds/muffin tin with cupcake liners and storage containers (mason jars are perfect for the storage of homemade lotions/body butters).

Before you move on to the next chapter and discover enticing recipes, one last word of advice. If you are going to use vitamin E oil as an ingredient, make sure you allow the mixture to cool down before adding it. Otherwise, all of its beneficial properties are going to disappear, the recipe being quite ruined. When used correctly, vitamin E oil can hydrate and repair damaged, dry skin.

Chapter 2 – Homemade lotions DIY recipes

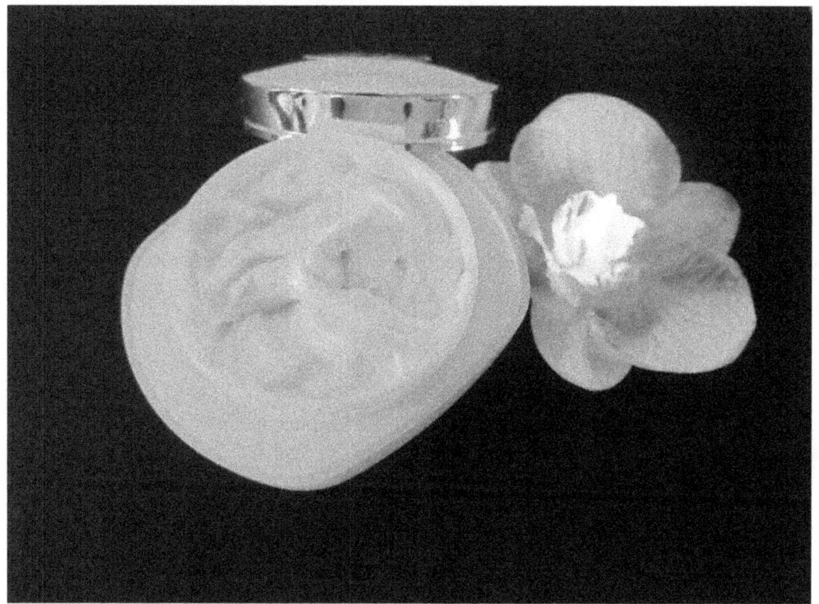

If you are interested in preparing nourishing lotions in the comfort of your own home, we have prepared no less than 15 DIY recipes you have to try out. As you will have the opportunity to read in the paragraphs that follow, these contain only natural ingredients. Follow the recommended steps and you will not have any difficulties in making them.

#1 Moisturizing lotion

Ingredients: almond/olive oil (1/2 cup), coconut oil (1/4 cup), beeswax (1/4 cup), vitamin E oil (1 tsp.), shea butter/cocoa butter (2 tbsp.), essential oils/vanilla extract (1 tsp.)

How to prepare:

Take a glass jar and combine all of the ingredients together. Then, take a saucepan and fill it with water. For the next step, place the saucepan over medium heat and the jar in the water, with the lid screwed on loosely. You will see that, once the water temperature rises, the ingredients are going to melt in the jar. Wait until the ingredients have completely melted and then pour the resulting mixture into a storage jar.

Wait until it cools down and apply to the skin, as you would do with any store-bought lotion. This homemade lotion can be used for about six months from the preparation date. Interesting enough, you can use this lotion not only to hydrate the skin and prevent stretch marks, but also to treat diaper rashes in babies and eczema in adults.

#2 Shea body butter

Ingredients: shea butter (1/2 cup), jojoba oil (2 tbsp.), lavender essential oil (10 drops), rosemary essential oil (10 drops), carrot seed oil (3 drops), tea tree essential oil (3 drops)

Note: in the situation that you do not have jojoba oil available, you replace it with other skin-nourishing oils; some of the greatest choices include olive, avocado, coconut, almond or apricot oil.

How to prepare:

After you have gathered all of your ingredients, take a saucepan and place it over medium heat. Add the shea butter and wait until it melts; then, add the jojoba oil and turn off the heat. For the next step, you will have to pour the resulting mixture into a bowl and place it in the freezer, in order to cool.

 Make sure that you keep the mixture in the freezer only about 15 minutes, so it becomes solid but not hard. Always remember that the mixture is not supposed to freeze.

When the recommended amount of time has passed, all you have to do is add the rest of the ingredients (lavender, rosemary, carrot seed and tea tree oil). Mix well, until all of the ingredients are properly combined and you have obtained the desired cream-like texture.

Be careful not to mix too much, as you will ruin the whole recipe. When done, pour the lotion into a jar and store at room temperature. You can use this lotion for the entire body, face included.

#3 Key lime whipped body butter

Ingredients: coconut oil (1/2 cup), olive oil (1 tbsp.), aloe vera gel (2 tbsp.), lime essential oil (20 drops), lemon essential oil (20 drops)

How to prepare:

You can begin preparing this recipe by adding all of the ingredients into a mixing bowl. It is important not to melt the coconut oil, as you can whip it only if it is still solid. Whip everything together for a couple of minutes or until you reach the desired consistency. Then, transfer the resulting mixture into a glass jar and squeeze the lid as tight as you can. You can store the key lime body butter at room temperature or in the fridge (depending on the temperature you have in your own home).

As a side note, you should not use a blender for this recipe, as you will actually warm the coconut oil and modify its consistency (thus, it will not be possible for you to whip it). Also, if you notice that the coconut oil is too soft for whipping, you can place it in the freezer for a couple of minutes before going through with the recipe.

#4 Rejuvenating homemade lotion

Ingredients: cocoa butter (1/2 cup), shea butter (1/2 cup), Argan oil (5 ml), rosehip oil (10 ml), Frankincense (10 drops), vanilla extract (20 drops)

How to prepare:

For the first step, you need to melt the cocoa and shea butter. You can achieve that by filling a saucepan with water and placing it over medium heat. Then, add the cocoa and shea butter into a jar and place it in the water. When melted, remove from the water and continue with the rest of the steps. Or, if you want, you can use a food dehydrator for such purposes.

Add the rest of the ingredients to the melted butters and then transfer them into a mixing bowl. Once they are properly combined, transfer them into a storage jar and place in the fridge, in order to cool down. This rejuvenating lotion can be particularly useful after you have taken a shower or a bath, nourishing the skin and preventing dehydration.

#5 Vanilla bean body butter

Ingredients: raw cocoa butter (1 cup), sweet almond oil (1/2 cup), coconut oil (1/2 cup), vanilla bean (1)

How to prepare:

The first step of the recipe requires that you melt the raw cocoa butter and coconut oil. This is easily achieved by placing the two ingredients into a jar; then, take a saucepan and fill it with water. Place the saucepan over medium heat and the jar in the warm water.

Once the cocoa butter and coconut oil have melted, remove them from the heat and let them cool for about half an hour. For the next step, use a coffee grinder to grind the vanilla bean (as an alternative, you can use a food processor). Add the ground vanilla bean, together with the sweet almond oil to the cocoa butter and coconut mixture.

Then, place them in the freezer for about twenty minutes. For the final step, whip the mixture until you achieve the desired consistency. Transfer into a storage jar and store it in a cool place.

#6 Lavender & mint body butter

Ingredients: extra-virgin coconut oil (1/4 cup), shea butter (3/4 cup), dried calendula petals (2 tbsp.), dried marshmallow root (2 tbsp.), lavender essential oil (8 drops), peppermint essential oil (8 drops)

How to prepare:

Begin by melting the coconut oil and the shea butter in a pan, in the pre-heated oven. Once melted, add the dried calendula petals and marshmallow root. Mix everything until they are well combined and place them back in the oven. The herbs should be left to steep for a couple of hours. If you have noticed that the mixture has solidified in the oven, all you have to do is warm it on the stove and then strain the herbs.

Add the resulting oil into a jar and place it in the fridge, until it becomes solid but not hard. For the next step, whip the oil for half a minute, then add the essential oils and mix some more. Transfer into a storage jar and use it whenever you desire.

#7 Whipped chocolate body butter

Ingredients: cocoa butter (1/2 cup), coconut oil (1/2 cup), cocoa powder (2 tbsp.), vitamin E (1/4 tsp.)

How to prepare:

Like the other DIY recipes, you can begin preparing this recipe by melting the cocoa butter and coconut oil in a jar, which was previously placed in a saucepan with water (over medium-heat). Once melted, remove from heat and place the mixture in the fridge, until it becomes solid but not hard.

Using a stand mixer, whip the cocoa butter & coconut oil mixture (you should go for a light and fluffy texture). Once you have finished whipping, it is time you added the cocoa powder and vitamin E. Mix all of the ingredients together, until they are even combined. Transfer the mixture into a jar and store it at room temperature (you can use it for about six months).

#8 Magnesium body butter

Ingredients: coconut oil (1/2 cup), cocoa butter (1/2 cup), magnesium oil (1/4 cup), essential oils (10-15 drops)

How to prepare:

Using a water-filled saucepan, melt the coconut oil and cocoa butter into a jar (placed in the said saucepan). As an alternative to this melting method, you can use a double boiler. Once these two have melted, it is time to add the magnesium oil. When all of the ingredients are properly combined, remove them from the heat and allow to cool down.

You can even store them in the fridge, until they become firm but not solid. Use a hand mixer and whip the ingredients, stopping when you have reached the desired texture. For the final step, add the essential oils of your choice and whip everything for another minute. Transfer into a storage jar and use whenever you need a calming lotion.

#9 Summer lotion

Ingredients: raw Manuka honey (1/2 tbsp.), aloe vera (1/2 tbsp.), calendula oil (3 tbsp.), chamomile essential oil (10 drops)

Note: in the situation that you do not have chamomile essential oil available, you can replace it with lavender oil (or other essential oil for that matter)

How to prepare:

Take a glass jar and add all of the ingredients into it. It is important that the glass jar is very clean or even sterile, in order to guarantee the success of the recipe. For the next step, close the lid of the jar and shake well to combine the ingredients. You can transfer the lotion into a storage jar and store it in the fridge. Note: given the fact that you have used raw honey for the making of this lotion, it is recommended that you should not apply it to children who are under one year of age.

#10 Red grapefruit lotion

Ingredients: virgin coconut oil (1/2 cup), raw shea butter (2 tbsp.), pure almond extract (1/8 tsp.), red grapefruit zest (from one fruit), tapioca starch (2 tsp.)

Note: both the coconut oil and shea butter should be at room temperature, when you begin preparing the recipe

How to prepare:

Take a mixer bowl and add the following ingredients: virgin coconut oil, raw shea butter, pure almond extract and red grapefruit zest. Mix everything together for about half a minute.

Then, increase the mixing speed and continue for another four minutes. The desired texture is light and fluffy. For the final step, add the two teaspoons of tapioca starch and mix for another half a minute. Transfer into a storage jar and store it at room temperature (recommended to be used within a month).

#11 Aloe vera & mint lotion

Ingredients: grated beeswax (1/4 cup), coconut oil (1/2 cup), aloe vera gel (1/2 cup), peppermint oil (1/8 tsp.)

Note: the aloe vera gel should be at room temperature before you begin preparing the recipe

How to prepare:

For this recipe, you can begin by melting the beeswax and the coconut oil. Fill a saucepan with water and place it over medium heat. Add the grated beeswax and coconut oil into a jar, then place the respective jar in the water-filled saucepan.

Once these are melted, remove them from the heat and allow to cool down. If necessary, add the mixture into the fridge (until it becomes firm but not solid). For the next step, add the aloe vera gel and the peppermint essential oil, mixing until all of the ingredients are properly combined. Allow the entire mixture to cool for about an hour, then whisk it again for a couple of minutes (this will give it a fluffier texture).

#12 Cranberry body lotion

Ingredients: coconut oil (1/4 cup), shea butter (1 tbsp.), frozen cranberries (1 tbsp.), orange essential oil (1 drop)

How to prepare:

You can begin preparing this recipe, by adding the coconut oil and shea butter into a large bowl. Then, mix them with the help of a mixer, for a couple of minutes. Use a food processor to mash the frozen cranberries, then add them to the previous mixture.

For the next step, add the resulting mixture to a fine mesh sieve and press down on it with the help of a spatula. In this way, you will eliminate the cranberries pieces from the lotion. Add the orange oil to the cranberry mixture, making sure that everything is well combined. Transfer the mixture to a storage jar and use it whenever desired. You can keep it in the fridge and use it up to one week.

#13 Peppermint whipped body butter

Ingredients: coconut oil (1/2 cup), cocoa butter (1/2 cup), shea butter (1/2 cup), sweet almond oil (1/2 cup), vitamin E oil (1 tsp.), peppermint essential oil (2-4 drops)

How to prepare:

You can begin by melting the coconut oil, together with the cocoa and shea butter. This can be achieved by using a double boiler or by using a water-filled saucepan and a jar. Once they are melted 100%, remove from the heat and allow to cool. After they have cooled done, add the rest of the ingredients, meaning the sweet almond, vitamin E and peppermint oil.

Refrigerate for one hour or until it becomes firm (but not solid). Take the mixture out of the fridge and whip it, stopping when you have obtained the desired consistency. Transfer into a storage jar and use it whenever you desire (can be used between six and twelve months, depending on the room temperature).

#14 Rose water body lotion

Ingredients: sweet almond oil (1/4 cup), rose water (1 cup), beeswax (1 tbsp.), coconut oil (1/4 cup), cornstarch (1/4 cup), honey (5 tbsp.)

How to prepare:

Use a double boiler in order to melt the sweet almond oil, beeswax and coconut oil. Add another jar to the same saucepan and warm the rose water. Remove everything from heat and add all of the ingredients into a food processor.

Do not blend until all of the ingredients have cooled down (you will probably have to wait about twenty minutes). After that time has passed, blend at medium-speed and transfer the resulting mixture into a storage jar.

#15 Orange blossom & shea butter lotion

Ingredients: raw shea butter (10 tbsp.), organic orange blossom water (4-5 tbsp.), sweet orange essential oil (7-10 drops), grapeseed oil (1 tsp.)

How to prepare:

You can begin preparing this recipe by melting the shea butter and oils, using a double boiler. Once these have melted, remove from heat and allow to cool down. If necessary, you can place the resulting mixture into the fridge, until it becomes firm but not hard.

After 15 minutes, you remove the mixture from the cold and whip it with a mixer. The desired texture should be light and fluffy. After a couple of minutes, add the orange blossom water (gradually, not all at once) and keep on mixing. When done, transfer the lotion into a storage jar and use it whenever you desire.

Chapter 3 – Lotion bars recipes

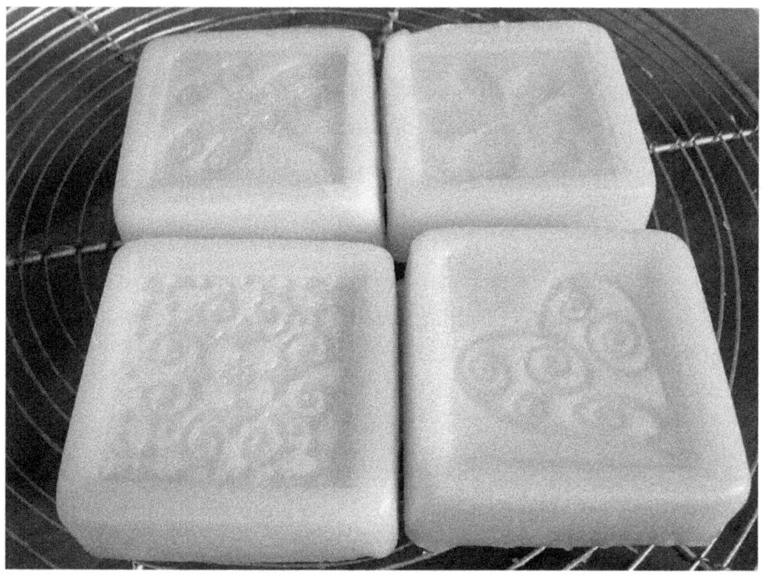

Photo source: Pixabay.com

Lotion bars can be easily prepared at home, just like the above-presented lotions and body butters. They provide the moisturizing effects of a lotion, being much more convenient to use in certain situations.

 As you will have the opportunity to see below, lotion bars require similar ingredients to lotions and body butter. Keep in mind that these lotions bars are going to melt for a little bit when coming in contact with your skin; in this way, they will moisturize and soften the skin.

#1 Orange & honey lotion bars

Ingredients: raw honey (1 ½ tbsp.), organic beeswax (4 tbsp.), organic shea butter (4 tbsp.), organic coconut oil (4 tbsp.), olive oil (1 tbsp.), organic orange essential oil (6 drops)

How to prepare:

Using a double boiler, melt the following ingredients: beeswax, shea butter and coconut oil. Make sure they are well combined and, once melted, remove them from the heat. Stir in the olive oil, honey and orange essential oil.

Take a muffin tin and place cupcake liners in each (preferably made from silicone). Place the muffin tin in the fridge, in order for the lotion bars to harden. You can also leave them to harden at room temperature but it will take a longer period of time.

#2 Coconut oil lotion bars

Ingredients: coconut oil (1 cup), beeswax (1 cup), shea butter (1/2 cup), almond oil (1/2 cup), lemon essential oil (6-7 drops)

Note: the beeswax can be grated or you can purchase it as pellets; as for the essential oil, if you do not have lemon available, you can replace it with lavender or rosemary oil

How to prepare:

Take a saucepan and fill it with water, then place it over medium heat. Add all of the ingredients into a glass jar and place it in the water (except for the essential oil). Mix from time to time, until all of the ingredients have melted and they are evenly combined. Allow the mixture to cool down before adding the essential oil, then pour it into silicone molds. You can leave it overnight to harden or place it in the fridge to speed up the process.

#3 Gold & Frankincense lotion bars

Ingredients: coconut oil (1/3 cup), shea butter (1/3 cup), beeswax (1/3 cup), gold mica powder (1 tbsp.), Frankincense essential oil (15 drops), Myrrh essential oil (15 drops), peppermint essential oil (10 drops; optional), lavender essential oil (10 drops; optional)

How to prepare:

Begin preparing this recipe by melting the coconut oil, shea butter and beeswax using a double boiler. Once these have melted and blended with one another, it is time to remove them from the heat. Allow the mixture to cool down before adding the gold mica powder and the chosen essential oils.

Mix everything to combine evenly and pour into silicone forms. You can leave the lotion bars to harden at room temperature or place them in the fridge for better results. Once they are done, you can rub them directly on the skin, in order to enjoy their moisturizing properties.

#4 Lavender lotion bars

Ingredients: beeswax (4 tbsp.), coconut oil (4 tbsp.), shea butter/cocoa butter (4 tbsp.), lavender essential oil (10-20 drops)

How to prepare:

Using a double boiler, melt the beeswax, coconut oil and shea butter/cocoa butter. As soon as they have turned liquid, it is important to remove them from the heat. Allow the mixture to cool down, then add the lavender essential oil and mix well to combine all of the ingredients. Pour the mixture into silicone molds and set aside to harden. If you want to speed up the process, you can place them in the fridge. When done, it is recommended to store them in a place that is cool and dry, otherwise they will melt.

#5 Chocolate lotion bars

Ingredients: coconut oil (3/4 cup), grated beeswax/beeswax pellets (3/4 cup), cocoa butter (1/2 cup), shea butter (1/4 cup), essential oils (20 drops), vitamin E oil (3 tsp.)

Note: you can choose any of the following essential oils – peppermint, lavender, lemon, orange and cinnamon

How to prepare:

You can begin preparing this recipe by melting the coconut oil, beeswax, cocoa and shea butter, with the help of a double boiler. Once these have melted, you can remove them from the heat. After they have cooled down, you can add the essential oils of your choice and also the vitamin E oil.

Mix everything well and then pour the resulting mixture into silicone molds. As with the other lotion bars, you can leave them on the counter to harden or, if you want, you can place them in the fridge.

Conclusion

The homemade lotions/body butters that you prepare in the comfort of your own home can be used on a daily basis, so as to hydrate and nourish your skin. If you customize the lotions, taking into account the skin type and eliminate the fragrances, you also use them for babies. While coconut oil remains a main ingredient for lotions, you can replace it with shea or cocoa butter, in order to create a nourishing body butter.

However, you must always take into account the skin type; for example, an oily skin does not require a body butter but rather a lightweight lotion. As for the dry skin, it might be more beneficial to apply a heavy body butter, that will hydrate and nourish it at the same time.

When you decide to try out making organic lotions, are taking a stand for yourself. You are finally saying goodbye to all those toxins that are used for the making of such products at an industrial scale. If you still not believe that this is true, just take your time and add all of the ingredients that are found in lotions, body butters and other similar products.

You will be amazed at how many toxins your body and your skin have to suffer from. With organic homemade lotions and body butters, you return yourself to simpler times. It is all about natural living and providing your skin with ingredients that are healthy and nourishing.

Making your own homemade lotion/body butter is even more essential if you have sensitive skin. Many of the store-bought skin care products can harm sensitive skin, leading to frequent irritations and redness.

If you are tired from always battling with such problems, you can use this book and create your own recipes. The good thing about these recipes is that they ensure diversity, which means that your skin will benefit from a wide range of nourishing products.

When we have so many natural ingredients available, why waste our money on store-bought lotions and body butters? It is time to make a change and begin preparing homemade skin care products. As for you, it is guaranteed you will have the time of your life while preparing these recipes, feeling enticed by all of those delicious scents.

Speaking about essential oils, it is worth mentioning that, apart from their wonderful fragrance, they also have antibacterial and antiviral properties. In conclusion, you can use them on your skin with all of the confidence, enjoying the added level of protection.

FREE Bonus Reminder

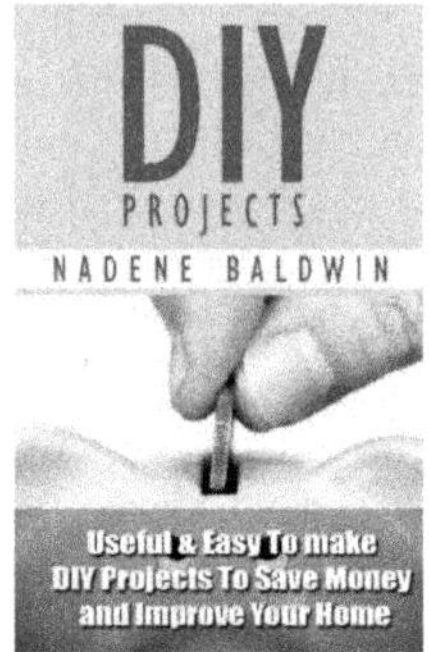

If you have not grabbed it yet, please go ahead and download your special bonus report *"DIY Projects. 13 Useful & Easy To Make DIY Projects To Save Money & Improve Your Home!"*

Simply Click the Button Below

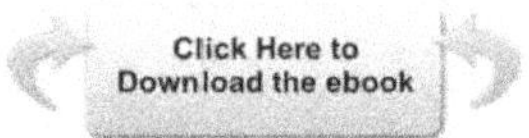

OR **Go to This Page**

http://diyhomecraft.com/free

BONUS #2: More Free & Discounted Books

Do you want to receive more Free & Discounted Books?

We have a mailing list where we send out our new Books when they go free or with a discount on Kindle. Click on the link below to sign up for Free & Discount Book Promotions.

=> Sign Up for Free & Discount Book Promotions <=

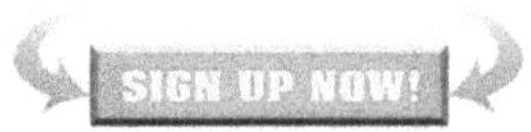

OR Go to this URL

http://zbit.ly/1WBb1Ek